BPD UNLOCKED

T.Z. Wiberg

Published by T.Z. Wiberg, 2026.

BPD UNLOCKED

First edition. July 6, 2026.

ISBN: 979-8235874749

Written by T.Z. Wiberg.

Table of Contents

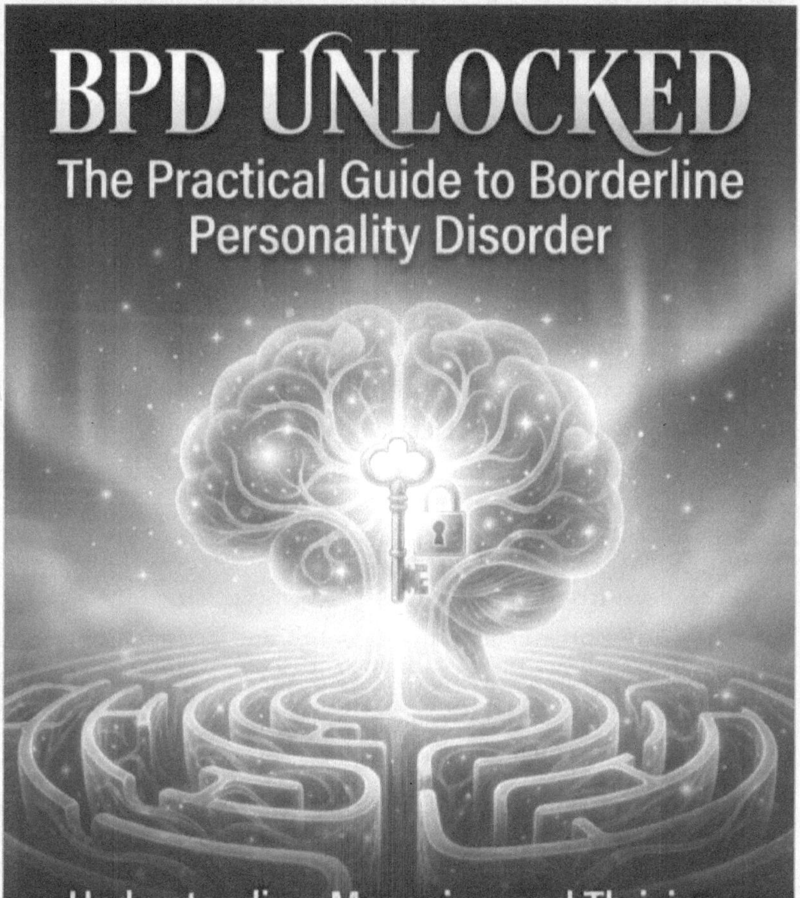
BPD UNLOCKED
The Practical Guide to Borderline Personality Disorder
Understanding, Managing, and Thriving.
Navigating Emotions and Building Stronger Relationships and Personal Growth.
The Introspective Guide to BPD:
A Personal and Practical Approach.
AUTHOR: T. Z. WIBERG

Introduction: The Key to the Labyrinth

If you are holding this book, you likely know the feeling: the internal storm that hits without warning, the intensity of emotions that feels like a language only you speak, and the exhausting, repetitive cycle of trying to navigate a world that doesn't seem to be built for the way your mind operates.

For fifty years, I have lived with the diagnosis of Borderline Personality Disorder. I have lived through the diagnostic labels, the trial-and-error of treatments, the stigma, and the profound, crushing weight of trying to understand myself in a world that often misunderstood me.

I am not writing this as a clinician observing from the other side of a desk. I am writing this as someone who has spent five decades inside the labyrinth.

This book is not a clinical manual meant to pathologize you. It is a roadmap born from my own lived experience, refined by the tools that actually made a difference in my daily life, and designed to help you reclaim your agency. The title *BPD Unlocked* isn't a promise of a cure; it is a promise of access. Access to your own emotional regulation, access to stronger connections, and access to a version of your life where the diagnosis is a context for your experience, not the ceiling on your potential.

I have spent a lifetime learning to dismantle the shame, navigate the volatile relationships, and build a structure that allows me to thrive rather than just survive. In these pages, I am handing you the key I found. It is a guide for the introspective, for the creators, for the feelers, and for anyone who is tired of being defined by the storm and is ready to learn how to navigate it.

We aren't going to talk about "fixing" you. We are going to talk about unlocking the potential you've always had, buried under the weight of an unregulated nervous system.

Let's begin.

Chapter 1 The Fundamentals
Part 1: The Labyrinth and the Label

For fifty years, I have been defined by a three-letter acronym: BPD.

If you look up "Borderline Personality Disorder" in most textbooks or scroll through internet forums, you will find a version of us that feels unrecognizable. You will see words like "manipulative," "attention-seeking," or "impossible." You will read about "volatile personalities" and "frequent interpersonal crises." To the outside world, this is a checklist of deficits. It is a portrait of a person who is fundamentally broken, someone to be managed rather than understood.

But that label is not who we are. It is a snapshot of our nervous system in a state of high-alert, taken by someone who doesn't understand the environment we are living in.

The Roots of the Storm

It is vital to be clear: BPD is not a random occurrence. For most of us, it is the deeply ingrained result of long-term trauma—often beginning in childhood. Whether through psychological or physical abuse, or a chronic invalidating environment, our brains were forced to adapt to survive.

The hyper-vigilance, the emotional intensity, and the difficulty in stabilizing our moods were not failures; they were brilliant, desperate adaptations to a landscape that was unsafe. Our brains learned to scan for threats and react with lightning speed because, at one point in our lives, that speed was necessary for survival.

The problem is that the environment changed, but the internal alarm system did not.

The Biological Reality: Emotional Sensitivity

At its core, BPD is a biological fact of extreme emotional sensitivity.

Imagine your nervous system is tuned to a frequency that is twenty decibels higher than everyone else's. A casual comment that might be background noise to an average person feels like a shout to you. A minor disappointment that others can brush off is, for you, a full-blown existential threat. This isn't because you are "dramatic." It is because your sensory input—emotional and environmental—is processed with higher intensity and a slower return to baseline.

Clinically, we are measured by the DSM-5 criteria: the fear of abandonment, identity disturbance, impulsivity, emotional instability, and chronic feelings of emptiness. These are the "symptoms" the world uses to label us. But when we look at them through the lens of trauma and sensitivity, they stop looking like personality defects and start looking like survival strategies gone into overdrive.

Navigation, Not Blame

The point of acknowledging this history is not to ride on the trauma or to use our damaged systems as a permanent excuse. Knowing *why* we are this way is simply the first step in recognizing that we are operating a complex, sensitive machine in a world that never provided us with a manual.

We cannot change the past that wired our brains this way, but we can learn to navigate the labyrinth it created.

We are not "difficult people"; we are people who have been operating with a faulty internal thermostat in a world that never taught us how to recalibrate it. You are not the label. You are the person who has been navigating a labyrinth with a blindfold on, and doing a remarkably resilient job of it for your entire life. Now, it's time to take off the blindfold and understand exactly how your mind works—not so you can be "fixed," but so you can finally learn to move through your life with the agency you deserve.

In the next section, we'll look at the physical, neurological reality of what happens when we experience "the storm."

Part 2: The Neuroscience of "The Storm"

When we talk about "the storm," we aren't using a metaphor for lack of a better word. We are describing a very specific, rapid-fire neurological event. When you live with the aftermath of long-term trauma, your brain becomes a master of threat detection, often at the expense of your own peace.

At the center of this is the amygdala—the brain's alarm system. For those of us with BPD, this alarm is exceptionally sensitive. It perceives a neutral facial expression, a slightly delayed text message, or a minor tone shift in someone's voice as an immediate emergency.

When that alarm goes off, the brain effectively "hijacks" our ability to think clearly.

- **The Physical Surge:** The moment the amygdala perceives a threat, it triggers a massive, instantaneous flood of stress hormones like cortisol and adrenaline. This is the "fight, flight, or freeze" response in overdrive, happening in a fraction of a second. You feel it in your body—the chest tightening, the heart racing, the sensation of heat rushing through your limbs, or the sudden, icy numbness that signifies "freeze."

- **The Prefrontal Cortex Shutdown:** Under normal conditions, the prefrontal cortex acts as the "brakes" of the brain—it is where we process logic, evaluate long-term consequences, and regulate our reactions. But during a storm, this part of the brain is essentially forced offline by the sheer volume of signals coming from the emotional centers. The "brakes" are cut, and your capacity for objective reasoning vanishes.

- **The Sensory Overload:** During the storm, the world itself can feel distorted. Colors might seem sharper, sounds more jarring. You lose the ability to maintain a balanced perspective because your brain is currently only programmed for one goal: surviving the immediate threat.

The Emotional Hangover

There is a profound, often misunderstood aftermath to these storms. After a period of intense emotion, you often feel a crushing weight of exhaustion, physical fatigue, and a deep sense of shame.

It is important to understand that this shame is not just a moral judgment you are making against yourself; it is the feeling of coming back online. As the prefrontal cortex begins to reboot and regain control, it looks back at the storm—at what you said, how you acted, or the intensity of your reaction—and experiences a kind of "buyer's remorse."

But this exhaustion is also neurological. You have just put your body through a high-intensity survival sprint. Your system has dumped a massive amount of energy into an emergency that, in reality, was likely not a life-or-death scenario. You are now paying the physical and emotional price for that energy expenditure.

Understanding this neurological cycle is crucial for removing the judgment. When you are in the middle of a storm, you aren't choosing to be irrational. Your prefrontal cortex—your seat of logic—has been temporarily locked out of the room by an alarm system that thinks you are in mortal danger.

The goal of our journey in this book isn't to get rid of the amygdala; it's to learn how to keep the prefrontal cortex involved even when the alarm goes off. It is about learning to recognize the first drops of rain so we can build shelter before the storm reaches hurricane force. You are not "broken" for having this response; you are simply operating with an alarm system that has been working overtime for a very long time, protecting you from threats that may no longer be there.

Part 3: Decoding the Checklist: A New Perspective on the Criteria

Most people who receive a BPD diagnosis are handed a piece of paper—a list of nine clinical criteria from the DSM-5. They are told to see if they meet at least five of them. For fifty years, I have seen these criteria used as a way to "prove" what is wrong with us. But after half a century of living this, I see them differently. These aren't signs of a broken personality; they are common pathways through a specific type of internal survival.

Let's look at the "official" clinical checklist through the lens of lived experience:

- **Fear of Abandonment:** It is called "pathological" in clinical books, but what if we call it what it is? It is a hyper-attunement to the safety of our most vital connections. When your early life taught you that people are unreliable or that connection is conditional, your brain learns to scan for exits constantly. It isn't a "fear"; it is a rational response to an unreliable world.

- **Identity Disturbance:** We are told we lack a "stable sense of self." But when you are forced to adapt your personality to survive different environments or different people from a young age, you become a master of reflection, not a person without a core. We don't lack a self; we have a self that has been hidden behind layers of protective camouflage.

- **Chronic Feelings of Emptiness:** This is often described as a "void." To me, it feels like the silence that follows a long, loud storm. It is the exhaustion of the nervous system when it finally has a moment to rest, and we mistake that quiet for a lack of meaning.

- **Impulsivity (in at least two self-damaging areas):** The clinician sees self-destruction. I see an attempt to regulate the nervous system. When the internal tension reaches a breaking point, we need a release. Impulsivity is often just a frantic, "quick-fix" attempt to lower the pressure inside the pressure cooker.

- **Recurrent Suicidal Behavior or Self-Harm:** This is the darkest part of the checklist. Clinically, it is a "symptom." In reality, it is the desperate, final protest of a soul that has not been given the tools to endure the intensity of its own reality. It is not a desire to end life; it is a desperate desire to end the *suffering* of the current moment.

- **Affective Instability (Emotional Swings):** This is the heart of the "storm." It is simply the result of an alarm system that cannot distinguish between a minor irritation and a major disaster.

- **Inappropriate, Intense Anger:** We are labeled "angry," but I have found that for us, anger is often the only emotion that feels "safe" to express because it creates distance. It is a boundary-setting tool that we never learned how to use in a healthy way.

Reclaiming the Map

When you look at this list, do you see a "personality disorder"? Or do you see a person who has been fighting to survive using the only tools they were given?

The DSM-5 criteria are just a description of the symptoms—they are the "what." But they never touch the "why." You now know the "why." You know about the trauma, the sensitive nervous system, and the hijacking of your prefrontal cortex.

You aren't a checklist. You are an individual who has been responding to a hostile environment with the best adaptation your brain could devise. We aren't here to check boxes; we are here to understand the mechanisms so we can finally start choosing our reactions instead of being ruled by them.

THE EMOTIONAL STORM CYCLE

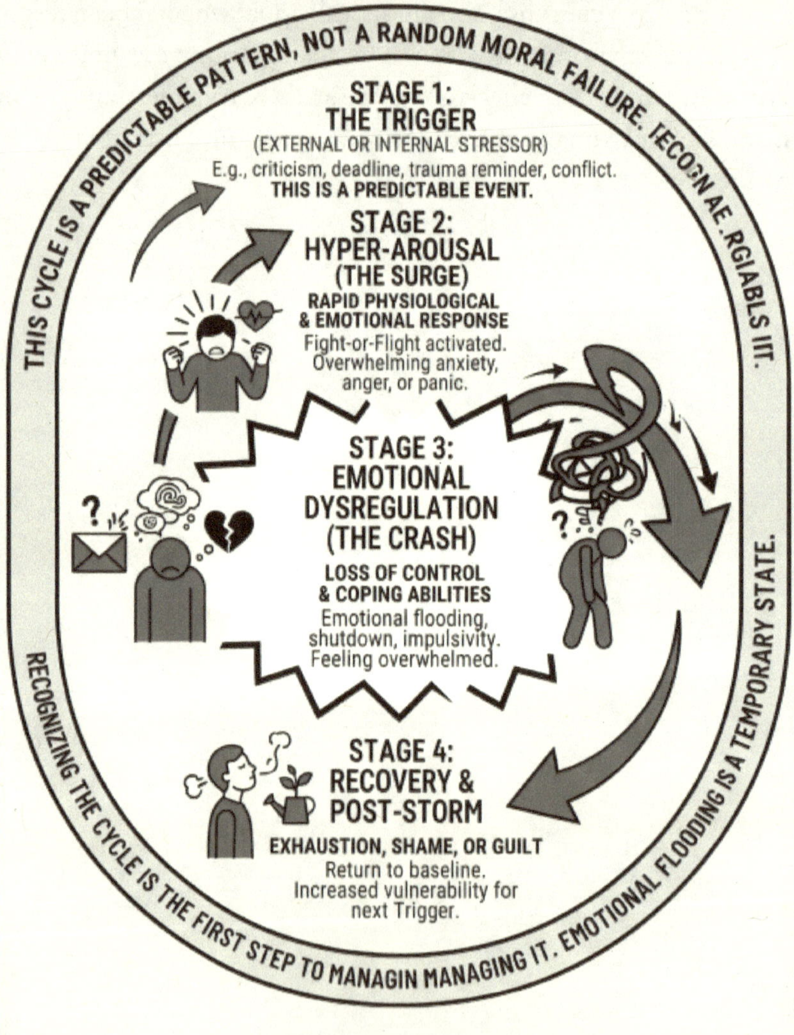

Chapter 2 Emotional Regulation Part 1: The Art of Surfing

If you have spent your life feeling like you are drowning in a storm, the idea of "emotional regulation" probably sounds like a cruel joke. In clinical terms, regulation is often described as the ability to maintain emotional stability. But for those of us with BPD, "stability" has always felt like a myth—a static, boring state that was perpetually out of reach.

When you hear "regulate your emotions," it is easy to hear "suppress your feelings." You might think it means clamping down on the intensity, forcing yourself to be calm when your blood is boiling, or acting like a person who doesn't feel a hundred things at once.

But that is not what regulation is. In fact, trying to force your emotions to stop is the fastest way to get crushed by them.

Learning to Surf

Think of your emotions like waves in the ocean. Some are small ripples, and others are towering, terrifying walls of water. When the big ones come, your first instinct is likely to fight them. You brace yourself, you tense your muscles, and you try to stand perfectly still against the force. And what happens? The wave hits you, tosses you, and pulls you under.

"Surfing" the wave is the opposite of fighting it.

Surfing is not about stopping the ocean from moving. It is about acknowledging that the wave is here, assessing its height and speed, and then adjusting your own posture so that you can ride it to the shore without being destroyed by it.

Regulation vs. Suppression

True emotional regulation is about agency, not control.

- **Suppression** is holding your breath and trying to push the wave away with your hands. It is exhausting, it is ineffective, and eventually, the wave wins.

- **Regulation** is acknowledging, "Okay, a massive wave is coming. I am feeling immense anger/sadness/fear right now. I am going to stay on my board, keep my balance, and ride this until the energy dissipates."

When we move from fighting our emotions to surfing them, the "storm" stops being a place where we go to die and becomes a place where we practice our balance. We stop asking, "Why am I feeling this?"—which is a question that often leads to shame—and start asking, "What is this wave teaching me about the current, and how can I stay upright while it passes?"

In this part of our journey, we are going to learn the technical skills—the balance, the stance, and the focus—that allow us to stop being the victims of the storm and start becoming surfers of our own lives. You don't need to be calm to be regulated; you just need to be present enough to stay on your board.

Part 2: The Witness at the Shore Developing the "Observing Self"

If mindfulness is about surfing, then the "Observing Self" is the surfer standing on the shore, watching the waves before they decide to paddle out.

For many of us, the hardest part of having a dysregulated nervous system is that we are constantly fused with our emotions. We don't just feel angry; we *are* anger. We don't just feel rejected; we *are* rejection. This fusion is what makes the storm feel so life-threatening—because there is no distance between "the storm" and "the self."

The goal of mindfulness in our context is not to "empty the mind." That's a tall order for anyone, and for a brain that scans for threats as a survival mechanism, it's practically impossible. Instead, we aim to cultivate what psychologists call the "Observing Self."

Creating Distance

Imagine you are sitting in a movie theater. On the screen, there is a horror movie playing. It's loud, it's terrifying, and the protagonist is in extreme danger. If you are deeply immersed in the film, your heart rate spikes, you hold your breath, and you might even want to run out of the theater.

But you are not the protagonist on the screen. You are the person sitting in the chair.

The "Observing Self" is your ability to move from being the protagonist in the horror movie to being the person in the chair. It is the part of you that can say, "Oh, look. My heart is racing right now. I notice my chest is tight. I am feeling a surge of fear because I think I'm being abandoned."

When you use the language of "I notice" or "I am aware that I am feeling," you are practicing the Observing Self. You are creating a tiny, precious gap between your raw experience and your identity.

Why the Gap Matters

This gap is where your freedom lives.

When you are fused with your emotions, you react reflexively. If you are scared, you lash out. If you are hurt, you withdraw. But when you are observing your emotions, you have options. You can decide: "I am feeling this intense wave of panic. Do I need to lash out, or can I just sit here and breathe while this wave passes?"

Developing the Observing Self doesn't mean you stop feeling the intensity—you will always be a deep feeler. It just means you stop being *blind-sided* by the intensity. You start to see the wave coming long before it hits, giving you the time to adjust your balance.

A Practice for the Overwhelmed

You don't need to spend hours on a meditation cushion to practice this. You can start right now, in the middle of your day. The next time you feel a shift—a spike of irritation, a pang of anxiety, a drop in mood—try these three steps:

- **Name it:** Use the phrase, "I am noticing that I am feeling [emotion]." (e.g., "I am noticing that I am feeling a sudden spike of anger.")

- **Locate it:** Where is it in your body? Is your jaw clenched? Is your stomach turning?

- **Validate it:** Remind yourself, "This is just a wave. It is a surge of chemicals, and it is a reaction to something I am perceiving.

I am the one observing it, and I am the one who can choose how to respond."

By observing, you aren't invalidating your feelings; you are honoring them by acknowledging them without letting them drive the bus. You are reclaiming the chair in the movie theater.

Part 3 Distress Tolerance: The Emergency Brake

If mindfulness is about maintaining your balance on the board, and the "Observing Self" is about watching the waves before they break, then Distress Tolerance is what you do when the wave has already crushed you.

There are times—we all know them—when the "Observing Self" feels like a distant fantasy. You are deep in the churn, the adrenaline is flooding your system, and the "storm" is at full hurricane force. In these moments, you don't need a meditation retreat; you need an emergency brake.

Distress Tolerance is not about fixing the problem, processing your childhood, or changing your personality. It is about one thing only: **surviving the crisis without making it worse.**

Radical Acceptance: The Power of "It Is What It Is"

The biggest trap we fall into during a crisis is the "Why is this happening to me?" loop. We fight the reality of the situation, which creates a second layer of suffering—the pain of *resisting* the pain.

Radical Acceptance is the practice of completely accepting reality as it is, without judgment or attempt to fight it. It doesn't mean you *like* what is happening. It means you stop banging your head against a wall and accept that the wall is there. When you say, "I am in the middle of a panic attack, and this is happening right now," you stop the secondary suffering that comes from wishing you were somewhere else. You stop fighting the wave and start allowing yourself to float.

The TIPP Skills: Changing Your Biology

When your prefrontal cortex is offline and the amygdala is screaming, logic won't save you. You need to hack your own biology to force your nervous system to downshift. DBT offers the **TIPP** skills for this purpose:

- **T - Temperature:** Splash ice-cold water on your face or hold an ice cube in your hand. The "dive reflex" is a biological trigger that forces your heart rate to slow down. It is a physical override button.

- **I - Intense Exercise:** Do something that uses all that "fight" energy. Run in place, do push-ups, or dance aggressively for sixty seconds. Burn off the adrenaline so your body doesn't keep pumping it into your brain.

- **P - Paced Breathing:** Slow your exhale down to be longer than your inhale (e.g., breathe in for 4 seconds, breathe out for 8). This signals to your parasympathetic nervous system that the threat is receding.

- **P - Paired Muscle Relaxation:** Tense a muscle group as hard as you can while you inhale, then release it completely as you exhale. This helps your brain distinguish between "tense and dangerous" and "relaxed and safe."

The "No-Damage" Rule

The goal of these skills is simple: survive the next hour without doing anything that will haunt you tomorrow.

Distress Tolerance is the art of buying time. When you are at a 10/10 on the intensity scale, you are incapable of making good decisions. By using these tools, you don't necessarily feel "better"—you just feel *less like a bomb.* You bring your intensity from a 10 down to a 7 or an 8, which is just enough space to let your rational mind back into the room.

You are not failing by needing an emergency brake. You are being responsible for the most sensitive, high-powered engine on the planet. Use the brake whenever you need it, and remember: the goal isn't to be perfect, it's just to get through the wave in one piece.

VISUAL GUIDE: THE TIPP SKILL TREE

CHAPTER 2, PART 3: THE EMERGENCY BRAKE

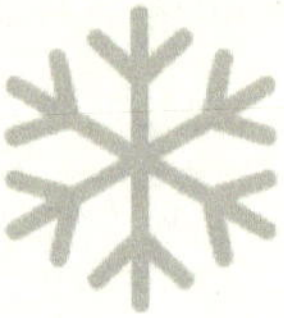

T: TEMPERATURE (Intense Cold)

Calms the sympathetic nervous system.

- Splash ice-cold water on face
- Hold a cold pack/frozen orange to eyes & cheekbones
- Lean forward, hold breath briefly.

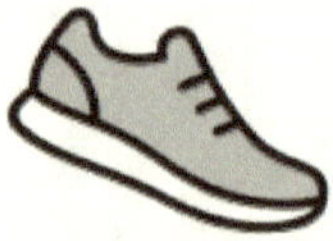

I: INTENSE EXERCISE

Burns off stress energy.

- Run in place for 2 minutes
- Do 20 jumping jacks
- Dance fast to music.

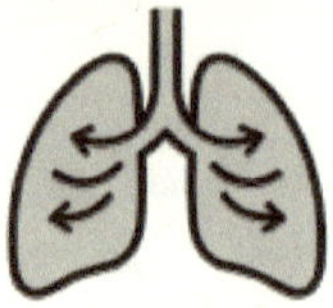

P: PACED BREATHING

Slows heart rate.

- Breathe in for 4 seconds INHALE
- Hold for 4 seconds
- Breathe out for 8 seconds (EXHALE icon).

4-4-8

P: PAIRED MUSCLE RELAXATION

Reduces overall tension.

- Tense muscles as you breathe in
- Relax muscles suddenly as you breathe out
- Focus on the feeling of release.

Part 4 Interpersonal Effectiveness: The Language of Boundaries

If surfing is your internal balance and the emergency brake is how you survive the crash, Interpersonal Effectiveness is the art of navigating the water with other people.

For many of us, relationships are the most dangerous part of the labyrinth. Because our nervous systems are so sensitive, we often interpret neutral interactions as threats, leading us to either "split" (seeing someone as all-good or all-bad) or withdraw to protect ourselves. Interpersonal effectiveness isn't about changing other people; it's about changing how you communicate your needs so you don't end up triggered or isolated.

The Power of the "Script"

When we are in the middle of an emotional wave, our communication usually becomes either passive (swallowing our needs) or aggressive (attacking to keep the "thteat" at bay). A script helps us bypass the emotional reaction and go straight to our goal.

Think of these as templates. They aren't meant to sound robotic; they are meant to provide a sturdy structure when your own prefrontal cortex feels flimsy.

1. The "I" Statement for Needs Instead of "You never listen to me," which triggers defensiveness in others and chaos in you, try:

"I am feeling [emotion] right now because [situation]. I would really appreciate it if we could [specific request]."

2. The Boundary Setter When you feel the urge to "split" because someone has disappointed you, buy yourself time to stay regulated:

"I am feeling very overwhelmed by this conversation and I don't want to react in a way that I'll regret. I need to take a break and process this, and I would like to come back to it in an hour."

3. The Validation Buffer Sometimes, others aren't giving us what we need, and that's painful. You can advocate for yourself without attacking:

"I understand you are stressed, but when you [action], I feel [emotion]. It's important to me that we find a way to communicate that doesn't feel like an attack."

Choosing Your Battles

Not every interaction requires a high-level script. Interpersonal effectiveness also means knowing which waves are worth surfing and which ones you can simply let pass. Ask yourself:

- **What is my objective?** Is it to be heard, to solve a problem, or just to keep the relationship stable?

- **Is my current intensity level appropriate for the situation?** If you are at an 8/10 on the intensity scale, *do not use a script yet.* Use your emergency brake first.

Communication is not about "winning" the interaction. It is about maintaining your dignity and your connection simultaneously. By having these scripts ready, you remove the guesswork. You stop reacting to the other person's behavior and start responding to the situation, which is a massive leap forward in maintaining your equilibrium.

You are learning to use your voice to set boundaries, not just to build walls.

CARE-MAP: THE CRISIS PREVENTION FLOWCHART

CHAPTER 2, PART 4: CRISIS PREVENTION

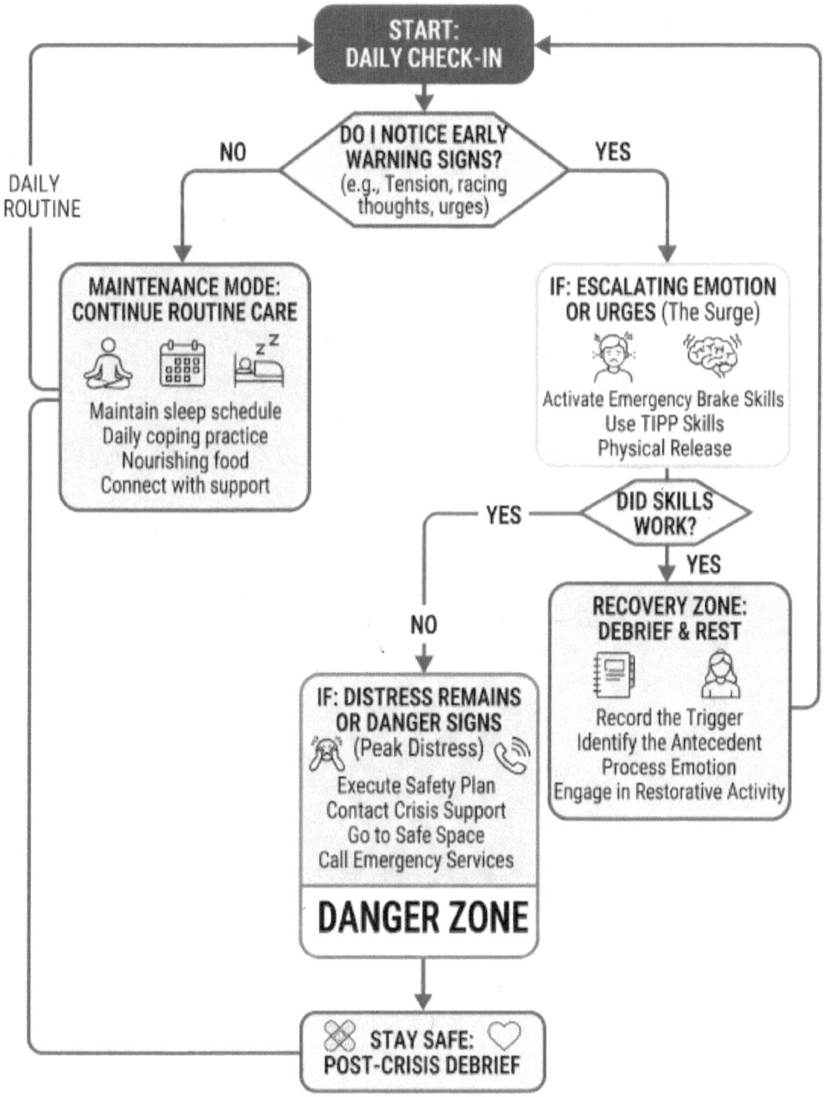

Chapter 3: Relationships
Part 1 Relationships and the Attachment Dance

If the "storm" is what happens inside our heads, then our relationships are the mirror that shows us what we fear most. For most of my fifty years, I viewed relationships through a binary lens: they were either my lifeline or my executioner. I didn't see people; I saw safety or I saw abandonment.

But there is a logic to this. When you have a history of trauma or a nervous system that perceives threats at double speed, you develop a specific style of attachment. You aren't just "needy" or "difficult." You are a person who learned to associate connection with potential loss.

The Attachment Dance

We often talk about "attachment styles" in clinical terms, but I prefer to think of it as a dance. Every relationship is a dance between two nervous systems. When you have BPD, your dance partner is usually a version of your past: a parent, a caregiver, or a former partner who proved that closeness was dangerous.

The "dance" usually involves two core maneuvers:

- **The Pursue:** When you feel the slightest hint of distance—a text not returned, a change in tone—your system goes into "pursue" mode. You reach out, you check in, you create noise to ensure the person is still there.

- **The Withdraw/Defend:** When you feel too much closeness, or when you anticipate hurt, your system goes into "withdraw" or "defend" mode. You pull back, you test the other person, or you lash out to create distance before they can leave you.

Most of us spend our lives alternating between these two steps, exhausted and confused, wondering why we can't just "be normal" in a relationship.

Seeing the Pattern

The first step toward healthier relationships isn't changing your partner. It is becoming aware of your own steps in the dance. Ask yourself:

- **What is my "Abandonment Trigger"?** What is the exact moment I stop being present and start "pursuing"? Is it silence? Is it a specific tone of voice?

- **What is my "Intimacy Trigger"?** When things are going well, when do I suddenly feel the urge to run, sabotage, or create a fight?

Recognizing these patterns is the beginning of the end of the "splitting" cycle. When you understand that your urge to push someone away is actually a survival mechanism—a way to avoid the perceived pain of future abandonment—you can stop identifying with the urge. You aren't "being mean" or "acting crazy." You are protecting a part of yourself that is terrified of being hurt.

The Goal: Stable Connection

We are not looking for relationships without conflict; we are looking for relationships where our nervous systems can feel "safe enough" to stay on the dance floor.

In this chapter, we are going to look at how to stop the frantic steps of the dance. We are going to explore how to set boundaries that protect your heart without closing it off, and how to stay connected even when your alarm system is telling you that the walls are closing in.

You are allowed to have needs, and you are allowed to be vulnerable. The goal is to learn how to do it without losing your sense of self in the process.

Chapter 3, Part 1

THE ATTACHMENT DANCE:

Understanding the Pursuer-Withdrawer Dynamic

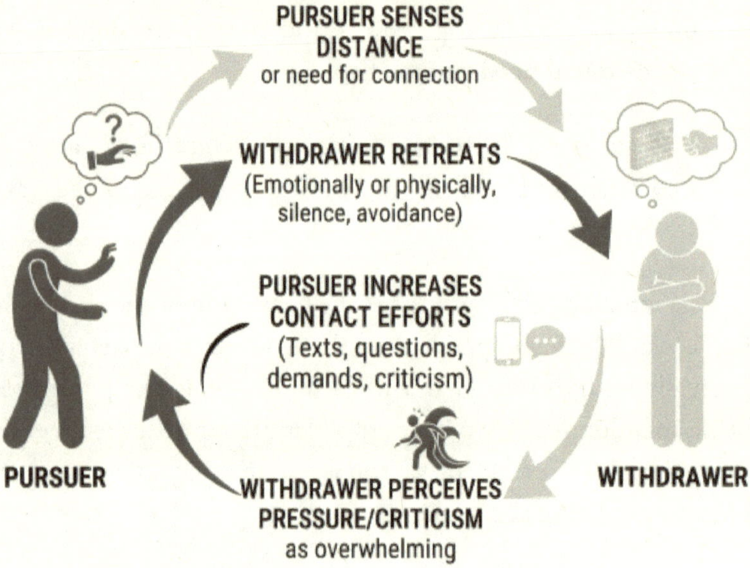

PURSUER'S CORE FEAR: BEING ABANDONED, UNIMPORTANT.
Seeks reassurance by pushing.

WITHDRAWER'S CORE FEAR: BEING FLAWED, CRITICIZED, FAILING
Seeks safety by retreating.

BREAKING THE CYCLE:
Recognizing the dance is the first step. Mutual vulnerability and understanding can shift the pattern.

Part 2 The Mechanics of Splitting: Seeing in Black and White

If the "Attachment Dance" is the rhythm of our relationships, "splitting"—clinically known as dichotomous thinking—is the breakdown of the music.

When we split, we lose the ability to see nuance. The person we love is either a saint, a savior, and the only person who truly understands us, or they are a monster, a traitor, and the source of all our pain. There is no middle ground. There is no "this person is a good friend who also happened to hurt my feelings today."

Why the Brain Splits

It is easy to label this as "drama." But in reality, splitting is a high-speed defensive maneuver.

When your nervous system perceives a threat—an act of rejection, a cold shoulder, a criticism—your brain effectively "reboots" your internal model of that person. If they hurt you, and they are supposed to be your "safe" person, that is a paradox your brain cannot handle in the heat of the moment. To protect you from the pain of that paradox, your mind takes a shortcut: *They aren't a safe person who hurt me; they are a bad person who was never safe at all.*

By shifting them to the "all-bad" category, you are trying to minimize the impact of the hurt. If they are "bad," their rejection matters less. You are essentially pre-emptively dumping them so they cannot dump you first.

The Internal "Reboot"

Splitting is a binary switch:

- **Idealization (The Saint):** You project all your hopes, needs for validation, and desires for wholeness onto this person. You make them responsible for your emotional stability.

- **Devaluation (The Monster):** When the inevitable human imperfection appears—when they forget to text back, when they are tired, when they have a bad day—the bubble bursts. Because you had placed them on a pedestal, the fall is catastrophic. The pedestal is smashed, and the "Monster" takes their place.

Catching the Split

The key to navigating splitting is realizing that **you are not seeing the person; you are seeing your reaction to them.**

To stop the cycle, you have to practice "dialectical" thinking—the ability to hold two opposing truths in your mind at the same time:

- "This person is capable of hurting me, and that is painful."
- "This person is still a human being with flaws who cares about me."

Try this the next time you feel the urge to "monster-ize" someone:

- **Pause:** Use your emergency brake skills. You cannot resolve a split while you are in a state of high emotional intensity.

- **Write it out:** Write down the "bad" thing they did, and then force yourself to write down two things they have done that were kind or supportive. It sounds simple, but it forces the prefrontal cortex to re-engage and acknowledge the "whole" person.

- **State the paradox:** Say to yourself (or even to them, if you are regulated enough), "I am feeling really hurt by what you did, and I am also having a hard time remembering that you care about me. I need to take a step back so I don't lose sight of the bigger picture."

You aren't trying to change your feelings; you are trying to bring the complexity back into the picture. Splitting thrives in the dark, binary corners of a crisis. Bringing in the gray areas—the "both/and"—is the light that breaks the spell.

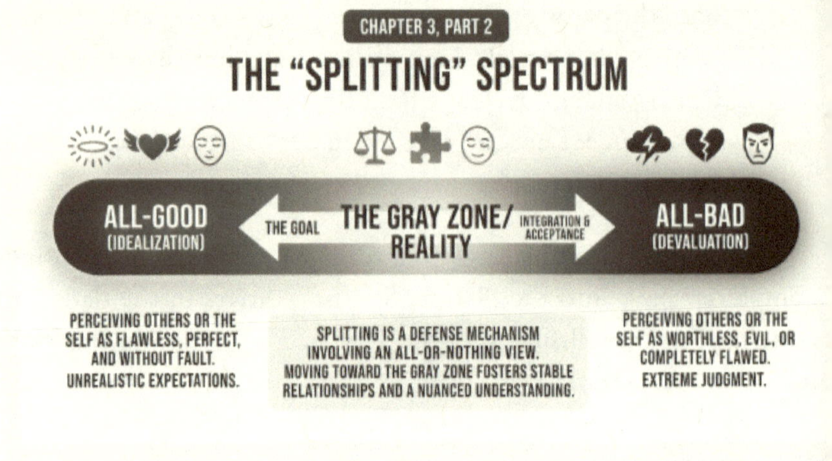
CHAPTER 3, PART 2
THE "SPLITTING" SPECTRUM
ALL-GOOD
(IDEALIZATION)
THE GOAL
THE GRAY ZONE/
REALITY
INTEGRATION & ACCEPTANCE
ALL-BAD
(DEVALUATION)
PERCEIVING OTHERS OR THE SELF AS FLAWLESS, PERFECT, AND WITHOUT FAULT.
UNREALISTIC EXPECTATIONS.
SPLITTING IS A DEFENSE MECHANISM INVOLVING AN ALL-OR-NOTHING VIEW.
MOVING TOWARD THE GRAY ZONE FOSTERS STABLE RELATIONSHIPS AND A NUANCED UNDERSTANDING.
PERCEIVING OTHERS OR THE SELF AS WORTHLESS, EVIL, OR COMPLETELY FLAWED.
EXTREME JUDGMENT.

Part 3 Setting Healthy Boundaries: From Walls to Gateways

If you have spent your life fighting the fear of abandonment, the word "boundary" probably sounds suspicious. You might associate it with exclusion, distance, or the precursor to someone leaving you. Many of us with BPD have lived with a "leaky" boundary system: we either let everyone in until we are depleted, or we build a fortress of walls to keep everyone out when we feel overwhelmed.

But a boundary isn't a wall. A wall is static, cold, and designed to keep people out permanently. A boundary is a gateway. It is a filter that allows the right kind of connection in while keeping your individual sense of self safe.

Why We Struggle with Boundaries

For us, boundaries are inherently tied to our attachment trauma. We often feel that if we say "no" or set a limit, the other person will view it as a rejection and walk away. We confuse *boundaries* with *abandonment*.

This is the fundamental distortion we have to correct. A healthy boundary doesn't reject the other person; it protects the connection. When you set a limit, you are actually preserving the relationship because you are preventing the resentment and burnout that inevitably happen when you over-give.

The "Flexible" Boundary

Think of your boundaries like the skin of your body. Your skin is permeable—it lets in oxygen and nutrients (connection, intimacy, care), but it keeps out harmful bacteria and viruses (disrespect, manipulation, overextension).

If your boundaries are too rigid (a wall), you starve the relationship of warmth. If your boundaries are too porous (a leak), you become vulnerable to infection and depletion. The goal is a boundary that is *firm but flexible.*

How to Build a Gateway

Setting a boundary is not an act of hostility; it is an act of self-preservation. Here are three ways to practice setting them without the panic of abandonment:

- **The "Time-Based" Boundary:** You don't have to address every emotional demand immediately. "I hear that you're upset, and I want to support you, but I'm currently at my capacity. Can we talk about this tomorrow morning when I'm feeling more centered?" This protects your nervous system while signaling that you are not "walking away."

- **The "Expectation" Boundary:** We often assume others should know what we need. When they don't, we "split." Instead, be explicit: "When I am feeling overwhelmed, I need twenty minutes of quiet time to reset. It doesn't mean I don't love you; it just means I need to regulate myself so I can be present with you."

- **The "Behavioral" Boundary:** This is about what you will and won't tolerate. "I want to have a productive conversation, but I cannot continue if there is shouting. If the tone remains aggressive, I am going to step out of the room until we can speak calmly."

The "Boundary Hangover"

When you start setting boundaries, you will likely feel a sense of "boundary hangover"—that familiar, gnawing anxiety that says, *"Oh no, I've done it now. They're going to leave me because I said no."*

When you feel this, remember: the people who truly care about you will respect your boundaries because they want you to be healthy and present. The people who get angry or try to punish you for setting a boundary are likely the ones who benefitted from you not having them.

Setting a boundary is the clearest way to see who is actually "in the dance" with you and who is just looking for a partner to control. You are not pushing people away; you are making room for the kind of connection that can actually last.

Part 4 Communication Scripts: The Tools for Connection

If boundaries are the gateway, then communication is the language we use to open them. For a long time, I thought communication meant *convincing* the other person to see things my way. I thought if I could just articulate my pain perfectly, they would finally understand, the threat would dissipate, and I could feel safe.

But communication isn't about winning an argument; it's about making sure you are both standing on the same reality. When you have BPD, your reality often feels like it's shifting under your feet. These scripts are designed to help you stabilize that reality so you can actually connect with the person in front of you.

The "I Feel" Formula

When we are triggered, we tend to lead with accusations: "You never," "You always," "You make me feel." These phrases are defensive walls. Instead, try the "I Feel" formula, which shifts the focus back to your internal experience:

> *"I feel [emotion] when [behavior] happens, because [the story I am telling myself]. What I need right now is [clear, actionable request]."*

- **Example:** "I feel anxious when you don't respond to my text for four hours because I start to worry that I've done something to push you away. What I need right now is for us to have a plan for when one of us is going to be busy, so I can soothe myself instead of spiraling."

The "I'm Flooded" Script

There is no shame in admitting you have reached your limit. In fact, it is the most respectful thing you can do for the relationship. When the "storm" is taking over, trying to force a conversation is like trying to do surgery in a hurricane.

> *"I can feel my nervous system getting overwhelmed. I am starting to feel like I'm going to split or say something I don't mean. I need to take 30 minutes to regulate, but I promise to come back and finish this conversation then."*

This script does three vital things: it sets a boundary, it explains the *why* (to avoid the other person assuming you are abandoning them), and it provides a concrete plan for reconnection.

The "Validation" Ask

Sometimes, you don't need a solution; you just need to feel seen. We often make the mistake of waiting for others to *guess* that we need validation.

> *"I am really struggling with [situation] right now. I'm not looking for a solution, but I would really value it if you could just tell me that I'm not crazy for feeling this way."*

Moving from Reaction to Response

Using these scripts requires a moment of pause—that "Observing Self" we talked about in Chapter 2. If you find yourself unable to use these scripts because the intensity is too high, *that is okay.* It just means you aren't in a place to communicate yet.

The goal isn't to be a master communicator overnight. The goal is to stop the reflexive, defensive firing that usually kills connection, and start using language that invites the other person into your world rather than pushing them away.

Relationships aren't meant to be survival situations. They are meant to be partnerships. By using these scripts, you are moving from a mode of "protecting myself" to a mode of "inviting connection."

Chapter 4 Lifestyle & Support
Part 1: Building Your Care Team

If Chapters 1 through 3 were about your internal architecture and how you relate to the world, Chapter 4 is about the scaffolding you build to keep the structure standing. For a long time, I thought "getting help" meant finding a professional who would tell me how to be "cured." I spent years in offices feeling like a patient waiting to be fixed by an expert.

But fifty years of living this has taught me a hard truth: You are the captain of this ship. Your doctors, therapists, and support staff are your crew. You are not a passive recipient of care; you are the manager of your own wellness.

Note: I am sharing what has worked for me throughout my journey. I am not a doctor, and this should not replace professional medical advice. Always consult with your own licensed healthcare providers regarding your specific needs.

The "Compatibility" Factor

Finding a therapist or psychiatrist who specializes in BPD is not enough. You need someone who speaks your language.

When you are interviewing a potential therapist, don't just look at their credentials. Look for:

- **The "Human" Element:** Do they seem comfortable with your intensity? If they look startled or clinical when you describe your "storms," they might not be the right fit. You need someone who can sit with the intensity without flinching.

- **The "Co-Pilot" Vibe:** A good therapist treats you like an adult. They don't just tell you what to do; they collaborate with you. They should respect your insight into your own brain.

- **Dialectical Fluency:** If they don't know the difference between "validation" and "agreement," or if they seem dismissive of the nuances of your trauma, be wary. You need a navigator who knows the terrain.

The Power of Firing Your Therapist

We are often taught to be "good patients"—compliant, quiet, and deferential to the doctor's authority. This is a trap. If you don't feel seen, if you feel judged, or if you feel like you aren't making progress, *you have the right to leave.*

Firing a therapist can be incredibly anxiety-inducing for us—it feels like a rejection, or like we are "quitting" on our own health. But it is actually a powerful exercise in boundaries. It shows you that you are the one in charge of your safety and your time.

Structuring the Team

A solid care team for BPD often looks like a three-legged stool:

- **The Therapist:** The one you work with on your "surf" skills, your attachment patterns, and your deep-dive trauma work.

- **The Psychiatrist/Prescriber:** Someone who understands that medication is about stabilizing the floor, not changing who you are. They should be willing to listen to your side effects and your lived experience with the meds.

- **The "Trusted Witness":** This doesn't have to be a professional. It is one person in your life—a partner, a friend, a mentor—who knows your signs of "splitting" or "going off-line." They aren't your therapist, but they are your early-warning system.

You are the CEO of your recovery. Build a team that listens to you, respects your expertise on your own life, and is willing to roll up their sleeves and get into the "storm" with you.

Placemet in **Lifestyle & Support**

Chapter 4, Part 1

CARE-MAP: THE CARE TEAM WHEEL

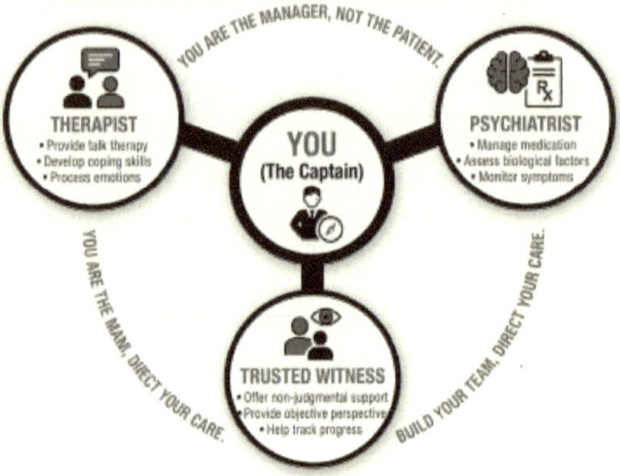

Part 2 The Safety Net: Your Personal Toolkit

Even the best care team cannot be with you 24/7. There will be nights when the storm hits at 3:00 AM, or afternoons when you are triggered in public and your therapist is unavailable. In those moments, you aren't just the captain; you are the engineer, the navigator, and the damage-control crew all in one.

Having a "Safety Net" isn't about being weak; it's about acknowledging that when your prefrontal cortex is offline, you shouldn't have to rely on your "thinking brain" to save you. You need a pre-programmed system.

The "Crisis Plan" (Before You Need It)

When you are in the middle of a surge, your brain loses its ability to organize and prioritize. This is why you should write your crisis plan while you are calm and "on-line."

Your crisis plan should be a simple, physical document (or a note in your phone) that answers these questions:

- **How do I know I'm spiraling?** List your early warning signs (e.g., "I start refreshing my emails," "I feel a cold, tight sensation in my chest," "I start thinking everyone hates me").

- **What are my "No-Brainer" Tasks?** If I am at a 10/10, what are three things I can do that require zero decision-making? (e.g., "Splash ice water on my face," "Call my sister," "Sit in the shower for 15 minutes").

- **Who is my "Emergency Contact"?** Is there one person you can call who won't try to "solve" it, but will just stay on the line?

Environmental Design: Hack Your Space

We often underestimate how much our environment dictates our nervous system. If you are prone to storms, your living space should be a "calm-down-zone."

- **Sensory Soothers:** Keep a physical basket in your home that is only for regulation. Put in things that engage your senses: a smooth stone (tactile), a specific calming scent like lavender (olfactory), a playlist of songs that are soothing (auditory), and perhaps a weighted blanket.

- **Remove the Triggers:** If you know that checking your social media feeds during a split causes you to spiral, make your phone "hostile" to that habit during high-stress times. Use website blockers or keep your phone in a drawer. You are not "censoring" yourself; you are protecting your nervous system from unnecessary over-stimulation.

The Power of Routine

For people with sensitive nervous systems, chaos is the enemy. Routine acts as an external scaffolding for your internal world. It doesn't have to be rigid, but having a "rhythm" helps.

If you know that waking up at a similar time, having a basic morning ritual, and going to bed with a "wind-down" process helps stabilize your baseline, do it. When you feel the storm coming, rely on the routine.

Don't try to come up with a brilliant, complex solution to your life. Just show up for the next hour of your routine.

The "Self-Care" Disclaimer

"Self-care" has become a buzzword, often associated with bubble baths and retail therapy. That is not what we are talking about here.

For the BPD nervous system, **self-care is maintenance.** It is the equivalent of checking the oil in a high-performance engine. It is about prioritizing your sleep, your nutrition, and your downtime *before* the crisis hits. You cannot pour from an empty cup, and you certainly cannot navigate a storm if you haven't slept in three days.

Building your safety net is an act of deep self-respect. It says, "I know I am vulnerable, and I know I have a sensitive system, so I am going to build a world that supports me."

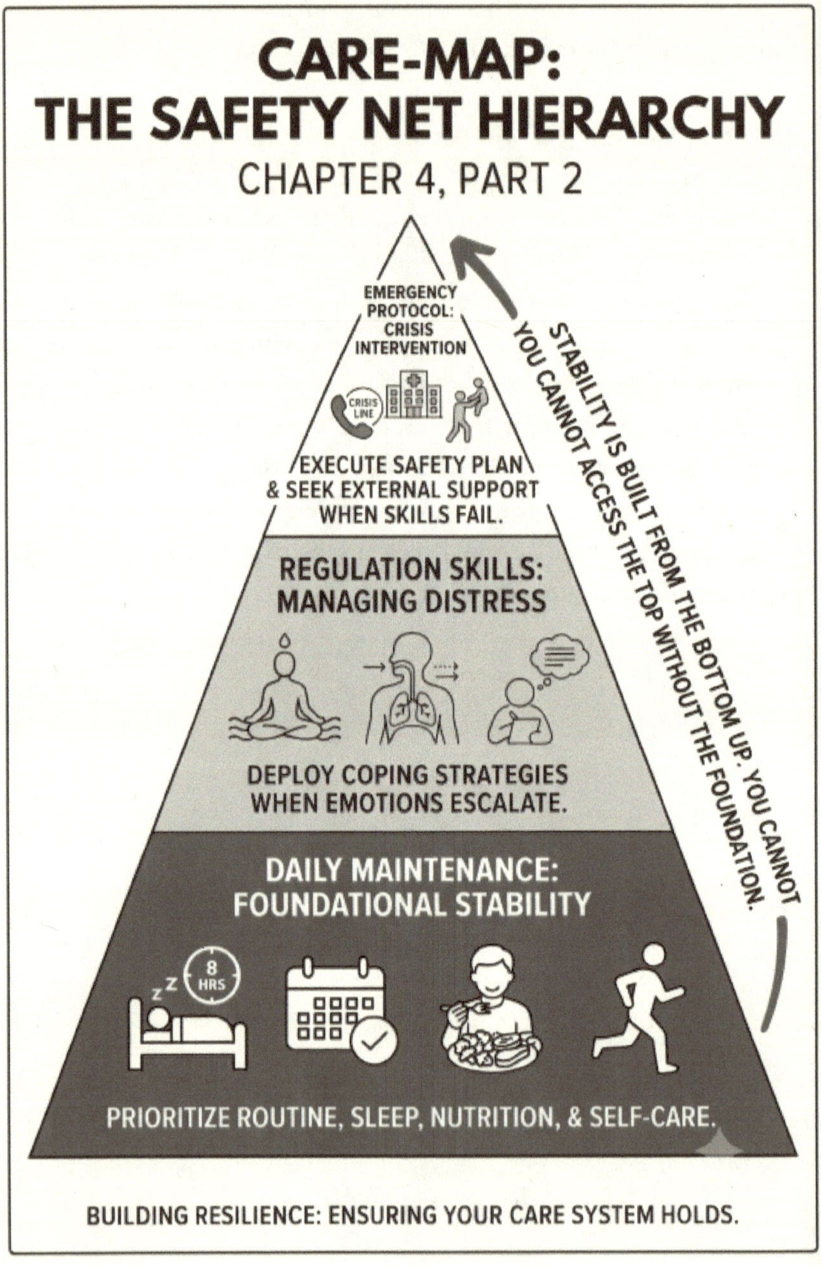
CARE-MAP:
THE SAFETY NET HIERARCHY
CHAPTER 4, PART 2
EMERGENCY PROTOCOL: CRISIS INTERVENTION
CRISIS LINE
EXECUTE SAFETY PLAN & SEEK EXTERNAL SUPPORT WHEN SKILLS FAIL.
REGULATION SKILLS: MANAGING DISTRESS
DEPLOY COPING STRATEGIES WHEN EMOTIONS ESCALATE.
DAILY MAINTENANCE: FOUNDATIONAL STABILITY
8 HRS
PRIORITIZE ROUTINE, SLEEP, NUTRITION, & SELF-CARE.
STABILITY IS BUILT FROM THE BOTTOM UP. YOU CANNOT
YOU CANNOT ACCESS THE TOP WITHOUT THE FOUNDATION.
BUILDING RESILIENCE: ENSURING YOUR CARE SYSTEM HOLDS.

Part 3: The Role of Medication
The Stabilizer: Medication and the Nervous System

Disclaimer: I am not a doctor, and I am not a psychiatrist. I am sharing my personal experience and the strategies that have worked for me. Please treat this as a conversation starter for you and your licensed healthcare team, not as medical advice.

For a long time, I resisted the idea of medication. I was afraid it would change who I was, or that it would "numb" the intensity that I felt was central to my creativity and my humanity. I wanted to "fix" myself through sheer willpower and therapy. What I learned the hard way is that you cannot do the work of therapy if your nervous system is in a constant state of hyper-arousal.

Medication for BPD is not a "cure." It is a stabilizer.

Raising the Floor

Think of your emotional life like a house. When you are in the middle of a BPD storm, the floor of that house feels like it's constantly dropping out. You are in freefall.

Therapy and mindfulness skills are like the furniture, the decoration, and the architecture of your house—they help you live well. But if the floor is missing, you have nowhere to put them.

Medication, in the right context, acts as a structural reinforcement. It doesn't tell you how to live, and it doesn't solve your trauma. It just keeps the floor from dropping out when the wind starts to blow. It raises your "baseline" of emotional stability just enough that you can actually hear your own thoughts again.

The "Volume Knob" Metaphor

I often tell people that my anxiety and emotional sensitivity feel like a radio that is permanently stuck at full volume. Every static crackle sounds like an explosion.

For me, the right medication didn't turn the radio off. I still feel the music, I still feel the heartbreak, and I still feel the joy. But it turned the volume down from a deafening 10 to a manageable 6 or 7. That difference—that little bit of extra room—is the difference between being overwhelmed and being able to choose how I respond.

The Reality of the "Trial and Error" Period

If you decide to explore medication, you need to be prepared for the "trial and error" phase. This is the part that isn't discussed enough.

Finding the right medication is a process of titration—finding that sweet spot where you feel stable but still "yourself." It can be frustrating. You might have side effects. You might try something that doesn't work. When this happens, do not view it as a failure of your "recovery." View it as an engineer testing different materials for the foundation of your house.

You are the CEO

Remember, you are the CEO of your care team (as we talked about in Part 1). The psychiatrist is a consultant. They provide the expertise on the chemistry, but *you* are the expert on the lived experience.

If a medication makes you feel "flat" or "robotic," speak up. If it's not touching the intensity, speak up. You are looking for a partner who listens to your report on how the medication is affecting your daily life and is willing to pivot until you find the right fit.

Medication is just one tool in your kit. It's not the answer to your life, but it can be the thing that keeps you upright while you find the answers for yourself.

Part 4 Finding Your Community: Breaking the Cycle of Isolation

For a long time, I treated my BPD like a state secret. I thought if I hid the intensity, the "splitting," and the messiness of my inner life, I could pass as "normal." The problem is that BPD thrives in silence. Shame feeds on isolation, and when you are the only one who knows the contents of your internal storm, you begin to believe the lie that you are "too much" or inherently broken.

Finding community is the antidote to that shame.

The Myth of the "Lone Warrior"

We often think that healing is something we do solo—that if we just read enough books, went to enough therapy, or practiced enough mindfulness, we would eventually "fix" ourselves. But BPD is a disorder of connection, and healing it requires connection.

When you find others who understand the landscape of your mind, something shifts. You realize that the "monstrous" thoughts you've been hiding are actually common human responses to extreme sensitivity. You realize you aren't an alien; you're just a person with a specific type of nervous system.

Healthy Community vs. Trauma Bonding

However, we have to be honest: not all "support groups" are helpful. There is a very real difference between *shared healing* and *trauma bonding*.

- **Trauma Bonding (The Trap):** This is when a group of people gathers to vent, obsess over their worst symptoms, and validate the idea that "nobody understands us except each other." It feels like relief in the moment, but it often reinforces the belief that the condition is unchangeable and that the outside world is inherently hostile.

- **Shared Healing (The Growth):** This is a community focused on *tools and thriving*. It's where you can say, "I am really struggling today," and the response isn't "Me too, let's wallow," but "I've been there; here is what helped me stay upright."

The difference is intention. Look for communities that focus on agency, recovery, and the "how-to" of living well, rather than just the "woe-is-me" of the symptoms.

How to Start Small

You don't need to join a giant, overwhelming group to start. Start with the "micro-community."

- **The "One-to-One" Connection:** Do you have one person in your life—a friend, a family member—who is capable of holding space without trying to "fix" you? Cultivate that relationship. That is your base camp.

- **Curated Spaces:** Look for peer-led support groups focused on DBT or mindfulness. These spaces are usually structured, which helps keep the nervous system regulated.

- **The "Parallel" Community:** Sometimes, the best community isn't a BPD support group at all. It's a hobby, a class, or a volunteer organization. Finding a space where you are defined by your *interests* rather than your *diagnosis* is incredibly healing for your sense of self.

The Courage of Being Seen

Moving beyond isolation takes immense courage. You are walking into a room (or a chat room) and saying, "This is who I am."

When you find that resonance—that moment where someone looks at you and says, "I understand exactly what you mean"—the shame evaporates. You stop being the "secret-keeper" and start being a human being again. Isolation is the cage; community is the key. You deserve to be heard, and you deserve to be supported by people who know that you are more than your diagnosis.

Chapter 5 For Loved Ones
Part 1: The Partner in the Storm

You Are the Anchor, Not the Doctor

If you are reading this, it means you care. You have likely spent nights wondering why things shifted so suddenly, why the person you love seems to react so strongly to minor events, or why it feels like you are constantly walking on eggshells. You have likely felt exhausted, confused, and perhaps even hurt by the sharp edges of their reactions.

I want to start by saying this, plainly and clearly: **It is not your job to "fix" them.**

The most common trap for loved ones of people with BPD is the "therapist trap." You start thinking that if you just love them enough, if you just say the right thing, or if you just prevent every possible trigger, you will save them from the pain. You might find yourself analyzing their childhood, tracking their triggers, or trying to provide logical solutions to their emotional spirals.

But when you take on the role of therapist, you cease to be a partner. You step into a hierarchy where you are the "healthy one" and they are the "broken one." This dynamic is not only exhausting for you, but it often triggers feelings of shame or inadequacy in your loved one, which ironically can lead to even more volatility.

BPD is a complex neurological and psychological experience. You cannot "love" the storm away, and you cannot "fix" a nervous system that is wired for hyper-vigilance. There is a profound difference between being a supportive partner and being a savior, and learning that distinction is the key to preserving both the relationship and your own sanity.

The Perspective Shift: From "Manipulation" to "Survival"

When you see your loved one lashing out, withdrawing, or shifting from intense affection to sudden hostility in a matter of minutes, it is easy to label this behavior as manipulation or malice. It feels personal because it happens to *you*, and it cuts deep.

But I want to offer you a different lens: **It is not about you.**

When someone with BPD "splits" or reacts with intense anger, they are not acting out of a calculated desire to hurt you. They are acting out of a state of internal terror. Their "threat alarm" has been triggered, their prefrontal cortex—the part of the brain responsible for logic, regulation, and empathy—has gone completely offline, and they are essentially fighting for their life in a room that is, to you, perfectly safe.

If you can stop seeing their behavior as a deliberate attack on your character and start seeing it as a sign of their *internal distress*, you will find the strength to remain the anchor in their storm rather than being pulled into it. You aren't being manipulated; you are witnessing someone lose their grip on their own reality.

Your Most Important Job: Presence

You don't need a degree in psychology to be a source of support. In fact, some of the most effective support is simple, quiet, and grounded.

- **Don't Fix; Hold Space:** When they are in the middle of a "storm," they don't need you to explain why they are wrong or why their reaction is illogical. Logic is the first thing to go in a crisis. Instead, use phrases like: *"I can see that you are in a lot of pain right now. I am here, and I am not going anywhere."* Your calm presence is more healing than any advice you could give.

- **The Power of the Boundary:** Supporting someone with BPD does not mean accepting abusive behavior. In fact, the most loving thing you can do for both of you is to set clear boundaries. If they are shouting, you can say: *"I care about you, and I want to hear what you have to say, but I cannot stay in this conversation if there is yelling. I'm going to go to the other room for 20 minutes so we can both calm down, and then we can talk."* This isn't abandonment; it's self-preservation that models healthy behavior.

- **Your Own Life is the Priority:** You cannot pour from an empty cup. If you sacrifice your mental health, your social life, or your own stability to "manage" your loved one, you are not helping. You are just creating two people who are burned out, resentful, and overwhelmed.

A Reflection for You

Being the loved one of someone with BPD requires a specific kind of strength. It is the strength to hold your ground while someone else is caught in a tidal wave.

You are not their therapist. You are not their savior. You are a person who loves them, and that is enough. You have your own needs, your own emotions, and your own life, all of which deserve to be nurtured. In the chapters that follow, we are going to look at the practical ways you can protect your own peace while continuing to be a supportive, grounded presence in their life.

Part 2 Understanding the Storm: Why They Lash Out (And Why It's Not About You)

If you are standing on the sidelines of someone else's BPD storm, it can feel like you are being held hostage. One moment, things are calm; the next, there is an explosion of anger, or a sudden, icy withdrawal, or a frantic plea for reassurance. It is deeply human to feel like the target of this behavior. It is natural to ask, "Why are you doing this to me?"

But here is the truth that will save your relationship: **When someone with BPD lashes out, they are not acting out of malice. They are acting out of terror.**

The "Threat Alarm"

Think of your loved one's brain as having a "threat alarm" that is permanently stuck in the *ON* position, a system that is constantly calibrated for a danger that most people never have to face. For most of us, an alarm is a discrete event that only screams when there is an actual, undeniable fire. It requires immediate, specific action. But for someone with BPD, that alarm is hyper-sensitive; it misinterprets neutral input as a catastrophic threat. It goes off if the toast is slightly burnt, if a text is delayed by ten minutes, if you shift your posture, or if you hesitate for a split second before answering a question.

When that alarm sounds, the physiological shift is total. Their prefrontal cortex—the sophisticated, rational command center responsible for logic, empathy, long-term planning, and emotional regulation—effectively goes offline. In that moment, they are not choosing to be difficult or irrational; they are literally losing access to the cognitive tools they need to navigate the situation calmly. They are no longer the person you know and love, because that "version" of them is temporarily inaccessible. They are, quite literally, in survival mode. Their nervous system is flooded with adrenaline and cortisol, screaming that they are under attack.

In this state of fight-or-flight, they are doing the only thing their biology knows how to do to escape the unbearable feeling of danger. They aren't trying to make your life difficult; they are trying to manage an internal emergency. They are lashing out to create a defensive distance, or they are clinging to you with frantic, desperate energy to ensure they aren't abandoned to whatever disaster they believe is unfolding. To them, the danger is as real as a physical threat, even if, from your perspective, everything in the room is perfectly safe.

The Myth of "Manipulation"

You have likely heard the word "manipulative" thrown around regarding BPD. I want to challenge that. Manipulation implies a calculated, cold-blooded plan to achieve a specific outcome.

What you are witnessing is not calculation; it is desperation.

When they try to provoke a reaction from you, they aren't trying to make your life miserable. They are trying to soothe their own unbearable internal pain. They are looking for *anything* that feels like a solid ground, and often, the only way they know how to find it is to test the boundaries of the relationship to see if you will stay. It's a tragic, self-defeating cycle, but it isn't an attack on your character.

What "Splitting" Looks Like from Your Side

When they "split" and suddenly treat you like the enemy, it feels like a slap in the face. But try to view it through this lens: You are the person they are most attached to, which means you are also the person they are most terrified of losing.

If they perceive that you might be pulling away, their brain tries to solve the pain by deciding you aren't safe anyway. It is a defense mechanism. They are trying to "devalue" you so that the impending (in their mind) abandonment hurts less. It is a shield made of anger, not a sword made of hate.

How to Stay Grounded

Understanding this doesn't mean you have to accept abusive behavior. It just means you don't have to absorb the blow.

- **Don't argue with the fire:** If they are in the middle of a "split" and accusing you of things that aren't true, do not try to win the argument. You cannot reason with a brain that is in survival mode. The more you defend yourself, the more "threatened" they feel.

- **The "I see you're in pain" approach:** When the storm hits, try to see past the words. Instead of responding to the accusation, respond to the emotion: *"I can see that you are really hurting right now, and I hate that you're feeling this way. I'm going to give us both some space, but I want to talk when things are calmer."*

- **Protect your reality:** You can acknowledge their pain without accepting their version of reality as the truth. You don't have to agree with their accusations to be supportive. You just have to be a steady, unshakeable presence.

Understanding that this is a *neurological storm* and not a *personal attack* is how you keep your own heart intact. You aren't being "got at"; you are witnessing someone struggling to navigate a reality that feels, to them, like a constant earthquake.

Part 3 Communication Rules: Navigating the Storm Without Losing Yourself

If you are a partner or loved one, you have likely been in a situation where the conversation spiraled into chaos. You try to use logic, you try to point out the facts, and you try to fix the misunderstanding—but the more you try, the more the argument intensifies.

When your loved one is in the middle of a "storm," their brain is in fight-or-flight mode. Their prefrontal cortex—the part that processes logic and nuance—is effectively offline. Trying to win an argument in that state is like trying to explain mathematics to a forest fire.

Here are the rules of engagement that will keep you from being pulled into the chaos.

Rule 1: Stop Trying to "Win" the Truth

When your loved one is splitting or experiencing a surge of intense emotion, they are not arguing about *facts*. They are arguing about *feelings*. If they say, "You never care about me!" and you respond with a list of all the things you did for them this week, you have missed the point. You are arguing the facts, while they are screaming about their internal experience of loneliness.

- **The Shift:** Instead of defending, validate the feeling. You don't have to agree with their version of the facts to acknowledge their pain.

- **The Script:** *"I can hear how painful this is for you, and I'm sorry you're feeling so alone. I want to understand what you're* *going through, but I'm struggling to follow when we're arguing about the past. Can we focus on how you're feeling right now?"*

Rule 2: The "Anchor" Technique (Don't Match Their Intensity)

If they are screaming, your instinct might be to scream back or to shut down completely. Both of these responses feed the storm. If you match their intensity, the fire grows. If you shut down, they feel abandoned.

Your job is to be the **Anchor**. An anchor does not fight the current; it stays firm, grounded, and unmoving. You can be the calm, consistent presence that remains after the storm settles. If you remain calm, you provide a model for them to mirror.

Rule 3: The Boundary as an Act of Love

Setting a boundary is not a punishment for them; it is a necessity for the relationship. If you allow yourself to be shouted at, you will eventually grow resentful. Resentment is the poison of long-term relationships.

- **The Script:** *"I care about you, and I want to hear what you have to say. But I cannot stay in this conversation if there is yelling. I'm going to go to the other room for 20 minutes so we can both calm down, and then we can talk. I'm not leaving you; I'm stepping away so we can have a better conversation."*

Crucial Note: You must follow through. If you say you are taking a break, take it. Do not use the time to brood; use it to regulate your own nervous system. When you come back, keep the conversation focused on the present.

Rule 4: Protect Your Reality

You can be supportive without adopting their version of reality as your own. You do not have to agree that you are "the worst person in the world" just because they are feeling a wave of intense anger and projecting it onto you.

Hold your own truth firmly. You can say: *"I know that's how you're feeling right now, and I'm sorry that it feels that way to you. But that isn't my reality, and I'm not going to agree to that narrative."*

The End Goal: De-escalation

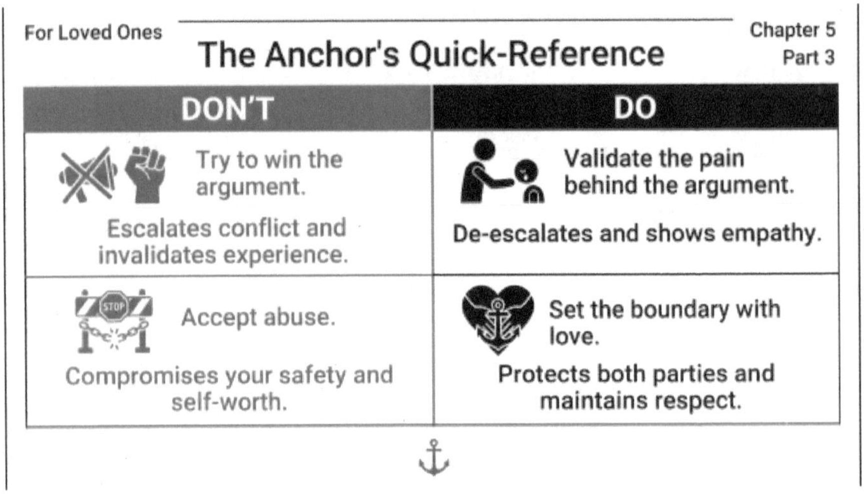

For Loved Ones — Chapter 5, Part 3

The Anchor's Quick-Reference

DON'T	DO
Try to win the argument. Escalates conflict and invalidates experience.	Validate the pain behind the argument. De-escalates and shows empathy.
Accept abuse. Compromises your safety and self-worth.	Set the boundary with love. Protects both parties and maintains respect.

Every interaction you have with your loved one is a choice. You can choose to enter the storm, or you can choose to stand on the shore and wait for the waves to settle. By refusing to engage in the "fight," you aren't being cold—you are being the partner they need. You are showing them that the relationship is stronger than the storm.

Part 4 The Anchor's Maintenance: Protecting Your Own Peace

If you have stayed with this chapter, you are likely the kind of person who cares deeply. You have been the listening ear, the calm voice in the storm, and the steady hand when everything else felt chaotic. But there is a dangerous trap that catches many of the best supporters: the belief that your own needs are secondary to the "crisis" at hand.

The role of an anchor is essential, but an anchor is not a martyr. If you let yourself become defined entirely by your loved one's emotional state, you stop being a partner and start becoming an extension of their disorder. That is not healthy for them, and it is catastrophic for you.

1. You Are Not the Savior

The most vital thing you can do for your loved one—and for yourself—is to let go of the idea that you are responsible for their "cure." You cannot love them "better," and you cannot save them from their own neural wiring.

When you stop trying to be the hero, a massive weight lifts. You aren't "giving up" on them; you are finally showing up as an equal. You are two human beings, not a savior and a patient. Accepting that their recovery is their own journey allows you to simply exist as a partner, which is the only thing that creates true intimacy.

2. Guard Your "Outside" Life

It is incredibly easy to let your world shrink until it only contains your loved one and their BPD. You might stop seeing friends because you're worried about what will happen if you leave, or you might skip your own hobbies because you feel guilty having "fun" when they are struggling.

This is the fastest path to resentment.

You must maintain your own identity. Keep your friends. Pursue your hobbies. Go on that trip. Your "outside" life is the source of your oxygen; it is where you recharge so that you have something left to give. If your life is vibrant and independent, you become a source of stability, not a hostage to the relationship.

3. The Resentment Early-Warning System

Resentment is the poison of long-term relationships. It doesn't appear all at once; it builds in the quiet moments when you say "yes" when you mean "no," or when you swallow your own needs to keep the peace.

- **Check-in with yourself:** Once a week, ask: *Am I feeling heard? Am I feeling used? Am I feeling energized or drained?*

- **Speak up early:** Do not wait for the resentment to boil over into an explosion. If something feels unfair, say it gently but clearly: "I really want to support you, but I'm feeling exhausted by [situation], and I need us to find a different way to handle this."

4. Build Your Own Support Network

Being the support person for someone with BPD is heavy lifting. You need your own space to vent, to process, and to be "the supported one."

- **Find a therapist:** Many partners of people with BPD find it immensely helpful to have their own therapist. It gives you a neutral place to unpack the stress, practice your own boundaries, and remember who *you* are outside of this relationship.

- **Don't keep it a secret:** While you should always respect your loved one's privacy, do not isolate yourself. Having friends who know the situation and can offer you a reality check is invaluable.

5. Final Reflection: The Healthy Mirror

Ultimately, you want to be a mirror that reflects the best of your loved one, not a sponge that absorbs the worst.

If you take care of yourself—if you stay grounded in your own reality, your own joy, and your own strength—you provide them with something far more powerful than "fixing": you provide them with the living proof that a stable, independent, and joyful life is possible.

You are an anchor, not a sacrifice. Keep your own light bright, and you will do more for them than any amount of "managing" ever could.

Thoughts on the road: The Alchemy of the Storm
A final word from the Author

Fifty years. When I look back at the map of my life, I don't see a straight line. I see a series of jagged, intense peaks and valleys. I have spent half a century living within the architecture of Borderline Personality Disorder, and if I am being entirely honest, there were years—many of them—where I felt completely crushed by the sheer weight of it.

There were times when the volume of my internal life was so deafening that I thought the only way to silence it was to disappear. The "storm," as we've called it throughout this book, is not a metaphor; it is a physical, visceral reality. It can take your breath, your relationships, and your sense of self in the blink of an eye.

But there is a strange, paradoxical truth to this life: the same intensity that nearly destroyed me became the vessel for everything I love most.

For a long time, I tried to "fix" the intensity. I wanted the volume turned down to zero. I wanted to be "normal." But over the decades, I learned that my sensitivity was not a flaw to be eradicated; it was an instrument to be played. When I stopped trying to kill the feeling and started trying to *channel* it, my world shifted.

My creativity became my salvation. As an author, an artist, and a musician, I found that the same brain that could spiral into darkness could also reach into the ether and pull down color, melody, and meaning. When I couldn't speak my truth to people, I painted it. When I couldn't handle the silence of my own head, I wrote into it. My creative life wasn't just a hobby or a profession; it was the mechanism by which I survived myself.

I have learned that the BPD experience is, in many ways, an experience of extreme depth. We feel the shadows deeply, yes—but we also feel the light in ways that others might never know.

If you are reading this, and you are currently in the thick of the storm, I want you to know this: You are not just a diagnosis. You are not a "patient." You are a person with an immense, terrifying, and beautiful capacity for feeling.

The path through this is not about becoming "empty" or "neutral." It is about becoming the architect of your own experience. It is about taking the intensity of your life and putting it to work—for you, rather than against you.

I still have days where the storm not only threatens to return, it crashes in like a tidal wave against the shore. I can face it fully aware of what it will do to me and those around me. But I am no longer the victim of it. I can, most of the time, handle the aftermath, and those around me understand and give me the space to bounce back. I also understand the impact it has from the other side. I cannot always stop the wave, but I can ride it like a surfer, and most of the time, navigate it.

I am the captain. And I have learned that even in the roughest waters, if you have your compass, your crew, and the courage to keep steering, you can navigate your way to something that feels like home.

You are more than the storm. You are the one who survives it, and in the aftermath, you are the one who gets to build whatever you choose.

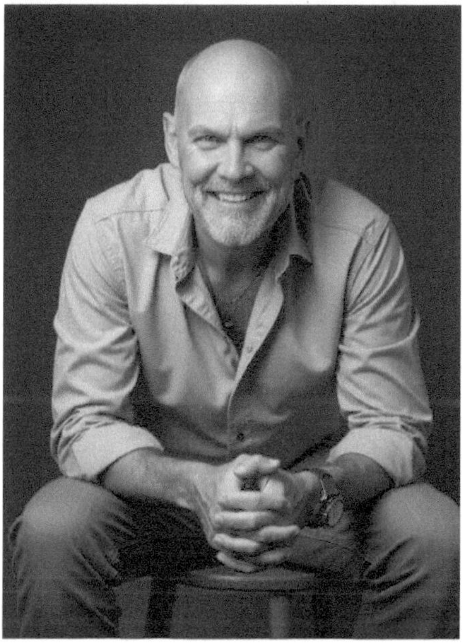

About the Author

I have spent fifty years living within the architecture of Borderline Personality Disorder, learning to navigate the storm rather than be crushed by it. As an author, artist, and musician, I discovered that creativity is not just a passion—it is the vessel of my own survival. I wrote this guide to share the key I found, hoping it helps you reclaim your own agency and build a life that finally feels like home.